The Complete Guide to Developing

NUTRITIONAL SKILLS

*The
ONE-STOP
Dietary Solution
for the Entire Family!*

Discover a Healthier Way to Live One Meal at a Time!

Delores D. Fedrick

PAGE PUBLISHING, INC.
New York, NY

First originally published by Page Publishing, Inc. 2015

ISBN 978-1-62838-904-3 (pbk)
ISBN 978-1-62838-905-0 (digital)

Printed in the United States of America

Acknowledgements

Thanks to the three hundred and thirty-two families from thirty-five churches throughout the South Carolina counties of Chester and York who participated in this initiative. Because of their commitment to health and wellness, the pilot study's outreach amassed more than three thousand participants from which the findings, successes, and lessons learned of this compilation are based upon. Special thanks to Reverend Angela W. Boyd and the congregation of the Metropolitan AME Zion Church in Chester, South Carolina, who served as a special twelve-week focus group. Their participation and efforts documented and further solidified the value of the principles of this manual.

Wholehearted and special thanks to Robert N. Fedrick, the illustrator and editor of the compilation.

Delores D. Fedrick

Preface

The need to understand proper nutrition is a national health emergency!

The American Medical Association and many medical professionals identify proper nutrition as the major determinant of health and wellness. The Centers for Disease Control and Prevention continue to report staggering rates of obesity as well as chronic diseases and their connection to unhealthy eating habits. All indicators point to improper nutrition as the insidious barrier to a healthy weight and improved quality of life. Yet, a Nielsen Global Consumer Insights poll revealed that the majority of Americans need easy-to-understand nutritional information to address this dire situation.

This guide delivers the essential, easy-to-understand nutrition toolset. Based on a grassroots initiative to provide a "universal" community nutritional solution, the resultant curriculum supplied the missing catalyst to raise public awareness of the diet-health relationship, the need for changed behavior, and the competence to do so. Through primary prevention, the program created awareness of the dietary risk factors that contribute to unhealthy weights, major chronic diseases, and causes of death. Detailing the predisposing, enabling, and reinforcing factors for health and wellness, the initiative created "knowledgeable dietary planners" and "lay nutritionists" who gained the skillset to take active roles in their families' health and wellness. The pilot group developed the toolset to choose diets that met individual nutrient requirements across age, gender, setting, family size, cultures, customs, and monetary resources. What's more, within the twelve weeks of instruction, the group developed the mindset to navigate through industrywide nutritional information effortlessly!

Therefore, this manual is written with a sense of urgency to share this "universal antidote" to the staggering nutritional crisis in America. It eliminates the need to consider more than 95% of the perplexing nutritional information that consumers are bombarded with daily. It responds to the need to involve every individual in their own nutritional requirements. The manual requires little to no initial guidance and demonstrates that, with a little practice, anyone and everyone can develop a thorough understanding of nutrition and thereby make personalized, smart, clear-cut, effortless, and affordable decisions about nutrition. The curriculum is transformative with instruction that can be retained equally well by children and adults. Moreover, the compilation fosters a mindset, toolset, and skillset of nutritional knowledge that can maintain any individual for life and not just for a few months or until one reaches an ideal weight.

The Complete Guide to Developing Nutritional Skills, considered by some to be an eye-opener for a real world need, can be used to assess current eating habits, and, if need be, choose diets that meet individual nutrient requirements, promote health, maintain healthy weights, support active lifestyles, and reduce the risks of chronic diseases. *The Complete Guide to Developing Nutritional Skills* is the *one-stop* nutritional and dietary solution for the entire family!

Introduction

Nourishment is a daily function that has become a daily task for most Americans! The goal of this compilation is to remove all of the difficulty and confusion. It provides the toolset to evaluate current eating habits and, if need be, make adjustments from that point. The manual is presented in levels with principles that can and should be committed to memory.

Level 1—Nutrition in Plain Language presents simple, clear-cut strategies to apply with each and every meal. It's all in plain language. There are no scientific expressions, just a base of general rules that can be easily understood so that eating healthier can begin immediately. (pages 9–17)

Level 2—The Real Answers in Nutrition decodes and simplifies the entire nutritional labeling system. **Level 2** is the backbone of this compilation, building an immediate bridge from one's current nutritional intake to the guidelines of public health experts. (pages 19–43)

Level 3—The Real Answers to Counting Calories builds on **Level 2**. For those who want to target counting calories, this level presents the tools necessary to accurately ensure the tracking of each and every calorie. (pages 45–53)

Level 4—Eat for Life builds on **Level 2** and provides the foundational skills needed to make shared decisions with medical professionals about chronic diseases including heart disease, diabetes, and certain types of cancers. (pages 55–65)

Level 5—Start Early! Age and Caloric Balance provides resources to fine-tune nutritional intake across age and gender, allowing appropriate caloric adjustments to be made during each stage of life. (pages 67–77)

Level 6—The Complete Nutrition Facts Label provides ready access to nutrient standards for every food component required for overall health. (pages 79–89)

Level 7—Reality Check! provides charts and goal setting tools to aid in determining current physical and medical status, and their alignment with the medical expectations of fitness. (pages 91–105)

Level 8—The 95% of Nutritional Claims That You Don't Need To Know! is provided for reinforcement purposes only. This level illustrates how the entire nutritional labelling system has been simplified by this compilation. (pages 107–115)

Reinforcement (page 117)

Use this manual to assess your current eating habits and, if need be, to choose diets that meet individual nutrient requirements, maintain healthy weights, address gaps in nutritional knowledge, and reduce the risks of chronic diseases.

LEVEL 1

Nutrition in "Plain Language"

With ten simple rules, Nutrition in "Plain Language" presents the most practical tools *in plain language* that an individual can use to maintain a healthy weight and good health in a timely and cost-effective manner.

Rule 1: When to Eat

Eat within one hour after waking up. Distribute meals and snacks at intervals of three to four hours throughout the day. Discontinue eating two to three hours before bedtime.

Rule 2: Nutrition At-A-Glance Plate Set-Up

There is a simple way to make quick yet informed food choices that contribute to a healthy diet. At every meal, at any setting (e.g., home, work, church, restaurants, or meetings), use the following straightforward rules:

1. The standard plate size is nine (9) inches! The plate size is important to control the size of your portions.
2. Make one-half (½) of your plate fruits and vegetables.
3. Rule 2 bears repeating! At every meal, make half your plate fruits and vegetables.
4. Make one-sixth (1/6) of your plate protein (i.e., poultry, fish, dry beans and peas, nuts, seeds, etc.).
   * A serving of meat is the size of a deck of cards!
   * Again, a serving size of meat is only the size of a deck of cards!!
5. Make at least one-fourth (1/4) of your plate grains, while making at least half of your grains whole grains (i.e., brown rice, oatmeal, whole wheat products, bulgur, English muffins, pita bread, bagels, tortillas, etc.).
6. Include a small side of dairy (fat-free/skim or low-fat/1% milk or yogurt).

Again, with all meals, whether they're eaten at home, a friend's house, work, church, restaurants, or civic and social gatherings, everywhere and every time, always follow the above plate design!

Source: www.ChooseMyPlate.gov

Rule 3: Fruits and Vegetables

As a follow-up to **Rule 2**, specifically numbers 2 and 3 above, special emphasis is given to fruits and vegetables because, daily, everyone should eat:

* Three (3) to five (5) servings of vegetables;
* Two (2) to four (4) servings of fruit.

Eating the daily requirement of fruits and vegetables is one of the most important choices an individual can make to help maintain a healthy weight and good health.

Choose different colors of fruits and vegetables to ensure optimal nutrition.

Vegetables and fruits are usually not packaged. Therefore, the serving sizes for vegetables and fruit follow:

A serving of vegetable is:

1 cup of raw leafy vegetables

½ cup of other vegetables, cooked or chopped raw

¾ cup of vegetable juice

A serving of fruit is:

1 whole (medium) fruit;

½ cup of sliced or cut-up fruit;

¼ cup of dried fruit;

¾ cup of 100% fruit juice

Reinforcement: See **Level 4 #5** - The Benefits of Eating Fruits and Vegetables (page 63).

Rule 4: Water

Although no single formula fits everyone, here are a few thoughts about water consumption:

* Drink eight (8) glasses of water daily, eight (8) ounces per glass;
* Replace surgery drinks with water;
* Drink water until the urine is clear.

Rule 5: Limit Added Sugar

The American Heart Association recommends limiting the amount of added sugars.

* For *women*, that's no more than 6 teaspoons or 24 grams of sugar per day;
* For *men*, that's no more than 9 teaspoons or 36 grams of sugar per day;
* For *children under 12*, that's no more than 3 teaspoons or 12 grams of sugar per day.

Reinforcement: 1 teaspoon = 4 grams (g)

More Reinforcement: Below are some products that have surprising amounts of sugar.

* One (1) Strawberry Yoplait Yogurt contains 27g of sugar!
* A can of Coca Cola has 39g of sugar! Would you eat 10 teaspoons of sugar or a stack of 10 sugar cubes?
* Eight (8) ounces of Mountain Dew contain 30g of sugar. That's more than 7 teaspoons of sugar!
* One (1) Kellogg's Pop Tart has 16g of sugar!
* Three Chips Ahoy Chocolate Chip Cookies have 11g of sugar. Who eats just three cookies?
* A pouch of Capri Sun has 16g of sugar, more than the daily recommendation for children under twelve!
* Eight (8) ounces of Minute Maid Orange Juice contain 24g of sugar!

Source: www.sugarstacks.com.

More Reinforcement: Read the ingredient list on food labels to determine if the product contains added sugars. Names for added sugars include:

Anhydrous dextrose	Brown sugar	Confectioner's powdered sugar
Corn syrup	Corn syrup solids	Dextrose
Fructose	High fructose corn syrup (HFCS)	Honey
Invert sugar	Lactose	Malt syrup
Maltose	Maple syrup	Molasses
Nectars	Pancake syrup	Raw sugar
Sucrose	Sugar	White granulated sugar

Source: www.ChooseMyPlate.gov

Nutrition Facts Labels don't list the amount of added sugars alone in a product. The line for sugars includes both added and naturally occurring sugars in the product.

Naturally occurring sugars are found in milk (lactose) and fruits (fructose). Any product that contains dairy (i.e. yogurt, milk, or cream) or fruit (fresh or dried) contains some natural sugars.

Rule 6: Watch Your Salt Intake

* An individual should consume only one teaspoon of salt (sodium) daily!
* Again, an individual should consume no more than one teaspoon of salt daily!

Rule 7: Limit Cholesterol

* An individual should not consume more than 300mg of cholesterol per day!
* One large egg has approximately 212mg of cholesterol!
* The yolk of the egg contains all the cholesterol.
* Cholesterol is only found in animal products.

Rule 8: Eating Slowly May Help

Digestion starts in the mouth. Chewing food thoroughly leads to better digestion. The more work the mouth does, the less work the stomach will have to do.

It takes the stomach about 20 minutes to produce the hormones that tell the brain that the stomach is full. The process does not start until the stomach begins to stretch. In slowing down, the stomach is given more time to start working on the food. It also allows more time to feel full.

By giving yourself more time to feel full, you'll improve digestion and the chances of stopping before "getting stuffed."

Rule 9: Eat Food, not Food-like Products!

* Eat foods that contain only one ingredient. It is what it is!
* Look for words like "raw," "sprouted," or "wholegrain." This indicates a more natural product.
* Avoid processed foods. The less processed a product is, the healthier it is.
* Eat a variety of healthful foods.

Rule 10: Drink in Moderation

According to the United States Dietary Guidelines for Americans, *moderate drinking* is defined as no more than one drink per day for women and no more than two drinks per day for men. Counted as one drink are the following:

* 12 ounces of beer
* 5 ounces of wine
* 1½ ounces of 80-proof hard liquor

Summary

This completes **Level 1**. Without addressing any of the complicated science around nutrition and food labeling, virtually anyone wanting to improve their nutritional intake will find that by applying these ten simple rules, they are eating to be healthy, eating to stay healthy, and/or eating to address health issues.

LEVEL 2

LEVEL 2

The "Real Answers" in Nutrition

Background: The Food and Drug Administration requires that the nutrient content of any food product be listed on the package's Nutrition Facts Label. When foods are not in packaged form, as is the case with fresh produce, Nutrition Facts Label information is displayed at the point of purchase (e.g., a sign, a binder, or another appropriate format in close proximity to the products).

All Nutrition Facts Labels are "based on a 2,000-calorie daily diet." Determined by the Food and Drug Administration, the 2,000-calorie benchmark has been found to be the "healthy" way to go for most consumers. All labels follow the same format, a list of substances called *macronutrients* and *micronutrients* (vitamins and minerals). (See pages 81 and 83). Macronutrients and micronutrients drive the body's metabolism, generate energy, prevent nutritional deficiencies, and help to avoid excesses in daily diets. This section will examine the macronutrients because they are the main determinants of health and wellness.

Overview: Here is the list of the major macronutrients that will be listed on a product's Nutrition Facts Label. This list is presented in the order in which these macronutrients appear on a label.

* Total Fat
    * Saturated Fat
* Cholesterol
* Sodium
* Potassium
* Total Carbohydrate
    * Dietary Fiber
    * Sugar
* Protein

Step 1: Getting Started

Familiarize yourself with the macronutrients and the numbers in red.

* Total Fat   65
    * Saturated Fat   20
* Cholesterol   300
* Sodium   2,400
* Potassium   3,500
* Total Carbohydrate   300
    * Dietary Fiber   25
    * Sugars
        * For women   24
        * For men   36
* Protein   50

These ten numbers, "the real answers", are the backbone of healthy eating for two important reasons:

* They are the daily targets or goals for each macronutrient of the 2,000-calorie-per-day diet.
* They give a thorough understanding of nutritional intake.

Each morning before breakfast, because you have not consumed any food, your body's lack of consumption of food is represented by the following Nutrition Facts Label.

Nutrition Facts
Serving Size

Amount Per Serving
Calories 0

	% Daily Values*
Total Fat 0g	0%
Saturated Fat 0g	0%
Trans Fat 0g	
Cholesterol 0mg	0%
Potassium 0mg	0%
Sodium 0mg	0%
Total Carbohydrate 0g	0%
Dietary Fiber 0g	0%
Sugars 0g	
Protein 0g	0%

*Percent Daily Values are based on a 2,000 calorie diet. Your Daily Values may be higher or lower depending on your calorie needs.

	Calories	2,000	2,500
Total Fat	Less than	65g	80g
Sat Fat	Less than	20g	25g
Cholesterol	Less than	300mg	300mg
Sodium	Less than	2400mg	2400mg
Total Carbohydrate		300g	375g
Dietary Fiber		25g	30g

Because you have not yet eaten, there are zeroes (0) beside each macronutrient. Note that these are the same macronutrients listed at the beginning of this section. (**Overview** on page 21)

By the end of the day, with the consumption of food, your body's Nutrition Facts Label should be represented by the following Nutrition Facts Label.

For Women

Nutrition Facts
Serving Size

Amount Per Serving
Calories 0

	% Daily Values*
Total Fat 65g	100%
Saturated Fat 20g	100%
Trans Fat 0g	
Cholesterol 300mg	100%
Potassium 3500mg	100%
Sodium 2400mg	100%
Total Carbohydrate 300g	100%
Dietary Fiber 25g	100%
Sugars 24g	
Protein 50g	100%

*Percent Daily Values are based on a 2,000 calorie diet. Your Daily Values may be higher or lower depending on your calorie needs.

	Calories	2,000	2,500
Total Fat	Less than	65g	80g
Sat Fat	Less than	20g	25g
Cholesterol	Less than	300mg	300mg
Sodium	Less than	2400mg	2400mg
Total Carbohydrate		300g	375g
Dietary Fiber		25g	30g

For Men

Nutrition Facts
Serving Size

Amount Per Serving
Calories 0

	% Daily Values*
Total Fat 65g	100%
Saturated Fat 20g	100%
Trans Fat 0g	
Cholesterol 300mg	100%
Potassium 3500mg	100%
Sodium 2400mg	100%
Total Carbohydrate 300g	100%
Dietary Fiber 25g	100%
Sugars 36g	
Protein 50g	100%

*Percent Daily Values are based on a 2,000 calorie diet. Your Daily Values may be higher or lower depending on your calorie needs.

	Calories	2,000	2,500
Total Fat	Less than	65g	80g
Sat Fat	Less than	20g	25g
Cholesterol	Less than	300mg	300mg
Sodium	Less than	2400mg	2400mg
Total Carbohydrate		300g	375g
Dietary Fiber		25g	30g

Because of your food consumption, there are now numbers beside each macronutrient. Note that these are the same macronutrients and numbers listed in red above (**Step 1** on page 21).

To simplify the Nutrition Facts Label even further, focus only on the portion of the Nutrition Facts Label circled below.

For Women   For Men

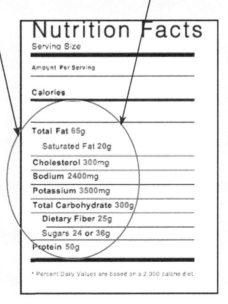

Note again that these are the same macronutrients and numbers listed in red at the beginning of this section (**Step 1**, on page 21).

Note that the only difference in the labels is the amounts of sugar, i.e. 24g for women and 36g for men.

These ten facts are the most important "facts" of the label. Therefore, from this point forward, all illustrations will reflect only this portion of the label, as shown below.

Step 2: Memorize the Ten Numbers

The ten numbers are the daily target amounts for each macronutrient of the 2,000-calorie-per-day diet.

* Total Fat   65
    * Saturated Fat   20
* Cholesterol   300
* Sodium   2,400
* Potassium   3,500
* Total Carbohydrate   300
    * Dietary Fiber   25
    * Sugars
        * For women   24
        * For men   36
* Protein   50

Step 3: Learn What the Ten Numbers Mean

These amounts mean that for a 2,000-calorie daily diet, when *all* of the numbers from *all* of the Nutrition Facts Labels from *all* of the foods that an individual consumes in one day are added together, the total amount for:

* Total Fat should not exceed 65
    * Saturated Fat should not exceed 20
* Cholesterol should not exceed 300
* Sodium should not exceed 2,400
* Potassium should be approximately 3,500
* Total Carbohydrate should be approximately 300
    * Dietary Fiber should be at least 25
    * Sugars (added) should not exceed:
        - For women—24
        - For men—36
* Protein should be at least 50

Following these macronutrient guidelines allows one to stay within the recommended 2,000-calorie-per-day diet.

You are now equipped with all the information needed, based on public health experts' advice, to effectively and efficiently drive the metabolism of the body. This is also the core of *The Complete Guide to Developing Nutritional Skills.*

Step 4: Example—Adding the Numbers

For breakfast, you have a bowl of cornflakes with a cup of milk and a banana. Read the Nutrition Facts Label found on each product below.

Cornflakes	Milk	Banana

Nutrition Facts	**Nutrition Facts**	**Nutrition Facts**
Serving Size · 1 cup	Serving Size · 1 cup	Serving Size · 1 small
Amount Per Serving	Amount Per Serving	Amount Per Serving
Calories 100	Calories 150	Calories 90
Total Fat 0g	Total Fat 8g	Total Fat 0g
Saturated Fat 0g	Saturated Fat 5g	Saturated Fat 0g
Cholesterol 0mg	Cholesterol 35mg	Cholesterol 0mg
Sodium 200mg	Sodium 120mg	Sodium 0mg
Potassium 45mg	Potassium 0mg	Potassium 360mg
Total Carbohydrate 24g	Total Carbohydrate 12g	Total Carbohydrate 23g
Dietary Fiber 1g	Dietary Fiber 0g	Dietary Fiber 3g
Sugars 0g	Sugars 0g	Sugars 12g
Protein 2g	Protein 8g	Protein 1g
* Percent Daily Values are based on a 2,000 calorie diet	* Percent Daily Values are based on a 2,000 calorie diet	* Percent Daily Values are based on a 2,000 calorie diet

Step 5: Add the Red Numbers

* Total fat from the cornflakes, milk, and banana labels:	0 +	8 +	0 =	8
* Saturated fat from the cornflakes, milk, and banana labels:	0 +	5 +	0 =	5
* Cholesterol from the cornflakes, milk, and banana labels:	0 +	35 +	0 =	35
* Sodium from the cornflakes, milk, and banana labels:	200 +	120 +	0 =	320
* Potassium from the cornflakes, milk, and banana labels:	45 +	0 +	360 =	405
* Carbohydrate from the cornflakes, milk, and banana labels:	24 +	12 +	23 =	59
* Dietary Fiber from the cornflakes, milk, and banana labels:	1 +	0 +	3 =	4
* Sugar from the cornflakes, milk, and banana labels:	0 +	0 +	12 =	12
* Protein from the cornflakes, milk, and banana labels:	2 +	8 +	1 =	11

So, for breakfast, you have consumed:

* 8g of Total Fat
* 5g of Saturated Fat
* 35mg of Cholesterol
* 320mg of Sodium
* 405mg of Potassium
* 59g of Total Carbohydrate
* 4g of Dietary Fiber;
* 12g of Sugar
* 11g of Protein

Step 6: Note the Serving Size

Find the location of the serving size circled below. The serving sizes for the cornflakes and milk are both one cup along with one (1) small banana.

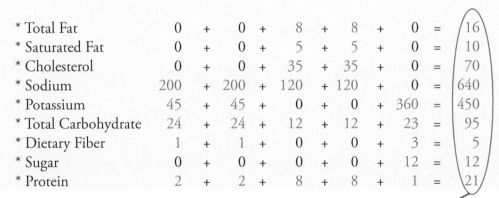

Cornflakes

Nutrition Facts
Serving Size   1 cup
Amount Per Serving
Calories 100

Total Fat 0g
  Saturated Fat 0g
Cholesterol 0mg
Sodium 200mg
Potassium 45mg
Total Carbohydrate 24g
  Dietary Fiber 1g
  Sugars 0g
Protein 2g

* Percent Daily Values are based on a 2,000 calorie diet.

Milk

Nutrition Facts
Serving Size   1 cup
Amount Per Serving
Calories 150

Total Fat 8g
  Saturated Fat 5g
Cholesterol 35mg
Sodium 120mg
Potassium 0mg
Total Carbohydrate 12g
  Dietary Fiber 0g
  Sugars 0g
Protein 8g

* Percent Daily Values are based on a 2,000 calorie diet.

Banana

Nutrition Facts
Serving Size   1 small
Amount Per Serving
Calories 90

Total Fat 0g
  Saturated Fat 0g
Cholesterol 0mg
Sodium 0mg
Potassium 360mg
Total Carbohydrate 23g
  Dietary Fiber 3g
  Sugars 12g
Protein 1g

* Percent Daily Values are based on a 2,000 calorie diet.

Reinforcement: If an individual has two cups of cornflakes with two cups of milk and one banana, then the addition becomes:

* Total Fat	0	+	0	+	8	+	8	+	0	=	16
* Saturated Fat	0	+	0	+	5	+	5	+	0	=	10
* Cholesterol	0	+	0	+	35	+	35	+	0	=	70
* Sodium	200	+	200	+	120	+	120	+	0	=	640
* Potassium	45	+	45	+	0	+	0	+	360	=	450
* Total Carbohydrate	24	+	24	+	12	+	12	+	23	=	95
* Dietary Fiber	1	+	1	+	0	+	0	+	3	=	5
* Sugar	0	+	0	+	0	+	0	+	12	=	12
* Protein	2	+	2	+	8	+	8	+	1	=	21

So for breakfast, the totals are:

* 16g of Total Fat
* 10g of Saturated Fat
* 70mg of Cholesterol
* 640mg of Sodium
* 450mg of Potassium
* 95g of Total Carbohydrate
* 5g of Dietary Fiber
* 12g of Sugar
* 21g of Protein

Step 7: Continue Adding the Nutrition Facts Labels for Everything Consumed throughout the Day

After having one cup of cornflakes, one cup of milk, and a banana for breakfast, you eat an apple. The Nutrition Facts Label for the apple is as follows:

Nutrition Facts

Serving Size 1 medium

Amount Per Serving

Calories 60

Total Fat 0g

Saturated Fat 0g

Cholesterol 0mg

Sodium 0mg

Potassium 103mg

Total Carbohydrate 17g

Dietary Fiber 2g

Sugars 14g

Protein 0g

* Percent Daily Values are based on a 2,000 calorie diet

Continue to add from **Step 5** on page 29.

*	8g of Total Fat	+ 0 =	8g of Total Fat
*	5g of Saturated Fat	+ 0 =	5g of Saturated Fat
*	35mg of Cholesterol	+ 0 =	35mg of Cholesterol
*	320mg of Sodium	+ 0 =	320mg of Salt
*	405mg of Potassium	+ 103 =	508mg of Potassium
*	59g of Total Carbohydrate	+ 17 =	76g of Total Carbohydrate
*	4g of Dietary Fiber	+ 2 =	6g of Dietary Fiber
*	12g of Sugar	+ 14 =	26g of Sugar
*	11g of Protein.	+ 0 =	11g of Protein

This is the total intake of macronutrients for the morning.

For lunch you have baked chicken, potatoes, and green peas. See the Nutrition Facts Labels below and continue to add the macronutrient amounts to the totals on page 33.

Chicken   Potato   Green Peas

Nutrition Facts
Serving Size   4 oz.

Amount Per Serving

Calories 210

Total Fat 15g
   Saturated Fat 4.5g
Cholesterol 90mg
Sodium 150mg
Potassium 0mg
Total Carbohydrate 0g
   Dietary Fiber 0g
   Sugars 0g
Protein 19g

* Percent Daily Values are based on a 2,000 calorie diet

Nutrition Facts
Serving Size   1 small

Amount Per Serving

Calories 50

Total Fat 0g
   Saturated Fat 0g
Cholesterol 0mg
Sodium 0mg
Potassium 300mg
Total Carbohydrate 12g
   Dietary Fiber 2g
   Sugars 1g
Protein 1g

* Percent Daily Values are based on a 2,000 calorie diet

Nutrition Facts
Serving Size   1 small

Amount Per Serving

Calories 60

Total Fat 0g
   Saturated Fat 0g
Cholesterol 0mg
Sodium 0mg
Potassium 180mg
Total Carbohydrate 10g
   Dietary Fiber 4g
   Sugars 4g
Protein 4g

* Percent Daily Values are based on a 2,000 calorie diet

Add the numbers:

*   8g of Total Fat   +   15.0   +   0   +   0   =   23.0g of Fat
*   5g of Saturated Fat   +   4.5   +   0   +   0   =   9.5g of Saturated Fat
* 35mg of Cholesterol   +   90.0   +   0   +   0   = 125.0mg of Cholesterol
* 320mg of Sodium   + 150.0   +   0   +   0   = 470.0mg of Salt
* 508mg of Potassium   +   0   + 300   + 180   = 988.0mg of Potassium
* 76g of Total Carbohydrate   +   0   +   12   +   10   =   98.0g of Carbohydrate
*   6g of Dietary Fiber   +   0   +   2   +   4   =   12.0g of Fiber
* 26g of Sugar   +   0   +   1   +   4   =   31.0g of Sugar
* 11g of Protein   +   19.0   +   1   +   4   =   35.0g of Protein

This is the total intake of macronutrients for breakfast, the morning snack, and lunch.

Continue to tally all the macronutrients from the Nutrition Facts Labels of the foods consumed for the remainder of the day.

For example:

*   After lunch, you have a cup of strawberry yogurt.
*   For dinner, you have roast beef, brown rice, corn on the cob, and brussels sprouts.
*   Later, you have popcorn.

The Nutrition Facts Labels for these food products follow on page 37.

Strawberry Yogurt

Nutrition Facts

Serving Size	1 container

Amount Per Serving

Calories 170

Total Fat 1.5g	
Saturated Fat 1g	
Cholesterol 10mg	
Sodium 85mg	
Potassium 230mg	
Total Carbohydrate 33g	
Dietary Fiber 0g	
Sugars 27g	
Protein 5g	

* Percent Daily Values are based on a 2,000 calorie diet

Roast Beef

Nutrition Facts

Serving Size	100g

Amount Per Serving

Calories 163

Total Fat 4g	
Saturated Fat 1g	
Cholesterol 54mg	
Sodium 39mg	
Potassium 0mg	
Total Carbohydrate 0g	
Dietary Fiber 0g	
Sugars 0g	
Protein 30g	

* Percent Daily Values are based on a 2,000 calorie diet

Brown Rice

Nutrition Facts

Serving Size	½ cup

Amount Per Serving

Calories 111

Total Fat 1g	
Saturated Fat 0g	
Cholesterol 0mg	
Sodium 5mg	
Potassium 0mg	
Total Carbohydrate 23g	
Dietary Fiber 2g	
Sugars 0g	
Protein 3g	

* Percent Daily Values are based on a 2,000 calorie diet.

Corn on the Cob

Nutrition Facts

Serving Size	1 medium

Amount Per Serving

Calories 80

Total Fat 1g	
Saturated Fat 0g	
Cholesterol 0mg	
Sodium 15mg	
Potassium 250mg	
Total Carbohydrate 17g	
Dietary Fiber 2g	
Sugars 3g	
Protein 3g	

* Percent Daily Values are based on a 2,000 calorie diet

Brussels Sprouts

Nutrition Facts

Serving Size	1 cup

Amount Per Serving

Calories 20

Total Fat 0g	
Saturated Fat 0g	
Cholesterol 0mg	
Sodium 15mg	
Potassium 230mg	
Total Carbohydrate 3g	
Dietary Fiber 2g	
Sugars 0g	
Protein 1g	

* Percent Daily Values are based on a 2,000 calorie diet

Popcorn

Nutrition Facts

Serving Size 2 tbsp unpopped/4 cups popped	

Amount Per Serving

Calories 180

Total Fat 12g	
Saturated Fat 2.5g	
Cholesterol 0mg	
Sodium 310mg	
Potassium 0mg	
Total Carbohydrate 15g	
Dietary Fiber 3g	
Sugars 0g	
Protein 2g	

* Percent Daily Values are based on a 2,000 calorie diet

When these macronutrient amounts are combined with the macronutrient amounts from page 35, the total for each macronutrient consumed for the entire day is:

* 42.5g of Total Fat
* 14.0g of Saturated Fat
* 189.0mg of Cholesterol
* 939.0mg of Sodium
* 1,698.0mg of Potassium
* 189.0g of Total Carbohydrate
* 21.0g of Dietary Fiber
* 61.0g of Sugar
* 79.0g of Protein

The day's Nutrition Facts Label is represented below.

Nutrition Facts

Serving Size

Amount Per Serving

Calories

Total Fat 42.5g

　Saturated Fat 14g

Cholesterol 189mg

Sodium 939mg

Potassium 1698mg

Total Carbohydrate 189g

　Dietary Fiber 21g

　Sugars 61g

Protein 79g

* Percent Daily Values are based on a 2,000 calorie diet.

Step 8: Evaluate the Day's Consumption of Macronutrients

Some thoughts on the day's consumption of macronutrients may include:

* The top of the Nutrition Facts Label lists macronutrients to limit (i.e., total fat, saturated fat, cholesterol, sodium) because they can have adverse effects on health if eaten in excess. Today's consumption is within the range of the macronutrients to limit (i.e., total fat, saturated fat, cholesterol and sodium) - not eaten in excess. See **Steps 1–3**, pages 21–27.
* Add any additional salt/sodium used during the day. Remember **Rule 6**, page 15.
* Consider adding beans, peppers, onions, mushrooms, lettuces, cucumbers, etc., as sources of the 3,500mg of potassium needed daily. See **Steps 1–3**, pages 21–27.
* The bottom of the Nutrition Facts Label lists macronutrients to get enough of (i.e., fiber and protein) because these macronutrients are beneficial to health. Consider adding coconuts, raspberries, pears, etc., as sources of the 25g of fiber needed daily. See **Steps 1–3**, pages 21–27.
* The amount of sugar includes some added sugar, which does not exceed the 24-gram limit recommended for women or the 36-gram limit recommended for men. See **Rule 5**, pages 13–15.
* Note any additional sugar from beverages. For each teaspoon of sugar, add 4 grams. See **Rule 5**, pages 13–15.
* Note the amount of water consumed. See **Rule 4**, page 13.
* Consider any bread eaten with meals.
* Count any other additives, i.e., butter added to the corn on the cob.
* Consumed three servings (banana, apple, strawberries) of fruit. The recommendation is two to four servings of fruit daily. See **Rule 3**, pages 11–13.

*   Consumed four servings (potato, green peas, corn, brussels sprouts) of vegetables. The recommendation is three to five servings of vegetables daily. **Rule 3**, page 11–13.

The Goal – The Ten Daily Targets

*Total Fat	65
*Saturated Fat	20
*Cholesterol	300
*Sodium	2,400
*Potassium	3,500
*Total Carbohydrate	300
* Dietary Fiber	25
* Sugars:	
- For women 24	
- For men 36	
* Protein	50

Reinforcement: If any macronutrient is not contained in a product, some manufacturers will not include it on the list. Other manufacturers will include the macronutrient(s) and zero (0) beside the item.

Step 9: Track All Foods Consumed Each Day

Track all food eaten daily by adding each food's nutritional values from the Nutrition Fact Labels. Compare the totals to the ten nutritional targets that you have memorized.

* Total Fat	65
* Saturated Fat	20
* Cholesterol	300
* Sodium	2,400
* Potassium	3,500
* Total Carbohydrate	300
* Dietary Fiber	25
* Sugars:	
- For women 24	
- For men 36	
* Protein	50

Step 10: Monitor and Adjust

Monitor, compare, and make adjustments to your daily diet. Find foods and methods of achieving the ten daily goals. Proper nutrition is about each person analyzing the food intake needed to achieve nutritional adequacy.

Remember to eat a variety of foods.

Summary

Level 2 decodes the entire complicated nutritional system into ten basic answers for proper nutrition. You are now equipped with all the knowledge needed to have a thorough understanding of basic nutrition!

Combine these ten daily targets with the straightforward rules of the **Level 1 Rule 2** plate "at-a-glance" design on page 11. Remember, with all meals, whether they're eaten at home, a friend's house, work, church, restaurants, or civic and social gatherings, everywhere and every time, always follow the plate design in **Level 1 Rule 2**.

(The information shown is based on a daily intake of 2,000 calories. You may need to consume a different calorie level depending on your age and gender. See **Level 5**, pages 67–77.)

LEVEL 3

The "Real Answers" to Counting Calories!

Level 2 presented the logic or *the real answers to proper nutrition*. This level presents *the real answers to counting calories.*

Step 1: You've Memorized the Ten Macronutrients and Numbers (Level 2 Step 2, page 27)

* Total Fat	65
* Saturated Fat	20
* Cholesterol	300
* Sodium	2,400
* Potassium	3,500
* Total Carbohydrate	300
* Dietary Fiber	25
* Sugars	
* For women 24	
* For men 36	
* Protein	50

Step 2: Only Three Macronutrients Generate Calories (circled below)

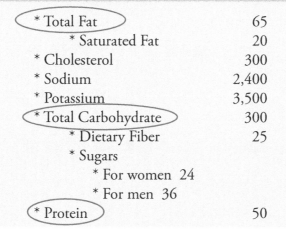

* Total Fat	65
* Saturated Fat	20
* Cholesterol	300
* Sodium	2,400
* Potassium	3,500
* Total Carbohydrate	300
* Dietary Fiber	25
* Sugars	
* For women 24	
* For men 36	
* Protein	50

Reinforcement: *Calories* are created from three sources or macronutrients:

1. Fats
2. Carbohydrates
3. Proteins

Step 3: Calculating Calories

To calculate calories or the amount of energy you get from food:

*   Multiply every fat gram (g) by nine (9)
*   Multiply every carbohydrate gram (g) by four (4)
*   Multiply every protein gram (g) by four (4)
*   Total the answers to get the total calories

Step 4: Note the Location of Calories on the Label

From the Nutrition Facts Labels that were shown in **Level 2 Step 4** on page 29 and also below, we see that 1 cup of cornflakes generates 100 calories, 1 cup of milk generates 150 calories, and a banana generates 90 calories, which comes to a total of 340 calories for breakfast.

	Cornflakes	Milk	Banana

Nutrition Facts (Cornflakes)
Serving Size .... 1 cup
Amount Per Serving
Calories 100
Total Fat 0g
  Saturated Fat 0g
Cholesterol 0mg
Sodium 200mg
Potassium 45mg
Total Carbohydrate 24g
  Dietary Fiber 1g
  Sugars 0g
Protein 2g
* Percent Daily Values are based on a 2,000 calorie diet

Nutrition Facts (Milk)
Serving Size .... 1 cup
Amount Per Serving
Calories 150
Total Fat 8g
  Saturated Fat 5g
Cholesterol 35mg
Sodium 120mg
Potassium 0mg
Total Carbohydrate 12g
  Dietary Fiber 0g
  Sugars 0g
Protein 8g
* Percent Daily Values are based on a 2,000 calorie diet

Nutrition Facts (Banana)
Serving Size .... 1 small
Amount Per Serving
Calories 90
Total Fat 0g
  Saturated Fat 0g
Cholesterol 0mg
Sodium 0mg
Potassium 360mg
Total Carbohydrate 23g
  Dietary Fiber 3g
  Sugars 12g
Protein 1g
* Percent Daily Values are based on a 2,000 calorie diet

Step 5: Calculating the Calories vs. Reading the Calories

Knowing how to calculate calories is very important in maintaining a healthy weight because manufacturers are allowed to round down the calories! To illustrate with the one cup of cornflakes, one cup of milk, and the banana from **Step 4** above and **Level 2 Step 5** on page 29:

*   8g of Fat ....8 × 9   =   72 calories
*   59g of Carbohydrate.....59 × 4   =   236 calories
*   <u>11g of Protein...............11 × 4   =   44 calories</u>

Total Calories   352 calories

Reinforcement: The Nutrition Facts Labels give the total calories (100 + 150 + 90) as 340. The exact calculation is 352 calories! This is one of the many reasons that everyone should understand nutrition. Manufacturers often round down the caloric content of products, which can mislead the consumer.

More Reinforcement: Calculating the calories for breakfast through lunch - **Level 2 Step 7** on page 35:

* 23.0g of fat	×	9	= 207
* 98.0g of carbohydrate	×	4	= 392
* 35.0g of protein	×	4	= 140
Total Calories		739 calories	

The Nutrition Facts Labels' total (100 +150 + 90 +60 + 210 + 50 + 60) is 720! Consider the amount of calories that are not counted if one relies on the Nutrition Facts Labels. The difference for an entire day can make a difference in maintaining a healthy weight.

More Reinforcement: Continue multiplying throughout the day
* Fat grams   ×   9
* Carbohydrate grams ×   4
* Protein grams   ×   4

Try to come as close as possible to the recommended amounts of the three macronutrients that create calories.

* Fat	65	× 9	=	585
* Carbohydrate	300	× 4	=	1,200
* Protein	50	× 4	=	200
				1,985 ≈ 2,000 calories

Calculating the total calories for the entire day (pages 37):

* 42.5g of Total Fat
* 14.0g of Saturated Fat
* 189.0mg of Cholesterol
* 939.0mg of Sodium
* 1,698.0mg of Potassium
* 189.0g of Total Carbohydrate
* 21.0g of Dietary Fiber
* 61.0g of Sugar
* 79.0g of Protein

* Fat	42.5g	×	9	= 382.5
* Carbohydrate	189.0g	×	4	= 756.0
* Protein	79.0g	×	4	= 316.0
				1,454.5 calories

More Reinforcement: Each gram of sugar in beverages (natural or added) should also be multiplied by 4 and added to the total calorie count for carbohydrates.

Summary

On a daily basis, track the caloric consumption for each family member. Don't forget about the plate "at-a-glance" design from **Level 1 Rule 2** on page 11. This will ensure that each person's intake is approximately 2,000 calories daily. Over time, you'll be able to make healthy choices without counting, tracking, or even thinking about it! After all, we are creatures of habit!

LEVEL 4

Eat for Life

Many of us do not appreciate good physical health until it is on the decline or we lose it to heart disease, cancer, diabetes, obesity, etc. Research has shown that certain diets raise the risk of developing these chronic diseases. Such diets are characterized by high intake of fat, cholesterol, and salt while the consumption of vegetables, fruits, and fiber is low. But many ask, "What is a high level of fat? How much is too much cholesterol? How much salt is too much? What is a high fiber diet?"

This section removes the generalities and gives "exact and plain language" answers to all these questions. It provides the basic toolset to make shared decisions with medical professionals. Knowing how to read food labels, illustrated in **Level 2**, is the foundation for developing the basic skills that are needed to address chronic diseases.

According to Emory University's School of Public Health's Eat for Life Program:

* To reduce the chances of getting certain types of cancer,
* To reduce the chances of getting heart disease,
* To prevent and control adult diabetes,
* To feel better physically,

Cook and eat healthy:

1. Reduce salt (sodium): You should consume no more than 2,000mg per day of salt.

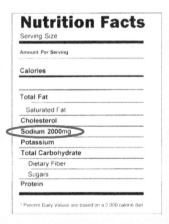

Caution: One teaspoon of salt is more than this!

For a 2,000 calorie daily diet, the amount of salt/sodium to be consumed for the entire day is 2,400mg or one (1) teaspoon. (See **Level 2 Steps 1–3**, pages 21–27).

But to reduce the incidence of certain types of cancer, heart disease, and adult diabetes, the recommendation is to decrease salt intake to 2,000mg per day. This 2,000mg of salt is less than one teaspoon per day!

2. Reduce cholesterol: You should not consume more than 300mg of cholesterol per day.

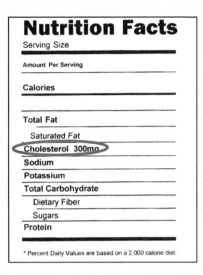

Caution: One large egg has 212mg of cholesterol!

Remember, the yolk of the egg contains all of the cholesterol. Cholesterol is only found in animal products.

3. Reduce total fat: You should consume 40–60g per day of total fat.

Nutrition Facts

Serving Size

Amount Per Serving

Calories

Total Fat 40g - 60g

Saturated Fat

Cholesterol

Sodium

Potassium

Total Carbohydrate

Dietary Fiber

Sugars

Protein

* Percent Daily Values are based on a 2,000 calorie diet.

Caution: One tablespoon of oil contains 14 grams of fat!

For a 2,000-calorie daily diet, the amount of total fat to be consumed for the entire day is 65 g. (See **Level 2 Steps 1–3**, pages 21–27.)

But to reduce the incidence of certain types of cancer, heart disease, and adult diabetes, the recommendation is to reduce the total fat intake range to 40–60g per day!

Start reducing fat by switching from solid fats to oils when preparing foods.

Examples of solid fats include:

* Beef, pork, and chicken fat
* Hydrogenated and partially hydrogenated oil
* Shortening
* Stick margarine

Examples of oils include:

* Canola oil
* Corn oil
* Cottonseed oil
* Olive oil
* Peanut oil
* Safflower oil
* Sunflower oil
* Tub (soft) margarine
* Vegetable oil

All vegetable oils are better for the body than animal oils/fat.

Source: U. S. Department of Health and Human Services.

4. Watch/avoid saturated fat. You should not consume more than 20g of saturated fat per day.

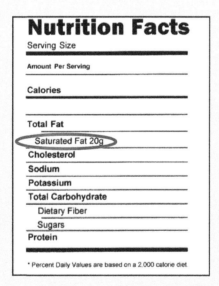

Caution: Limit intake of lard, meat, and other animal products!

For a 2,000-calorie daily diet, the amount of saturated fat to be consumed for the entire day is 20 g. (See **Level 2 Steps 1–3**, pages 21–27.)

There are two types of fat: saturated and unsaturated. Think of saturated fat as leaded gasoline. Think of unsaturated fat as unleaded gasoline. Just as most cars prefer unleaded gasoline, our bodies prefer unsaturated fat to stay healthy.

5. The Benefits of Eating Fruits and Vegetables:

Eat at least five (5) servings of fruits and vegetables every day. Diets rich in fruits and vegetables can:

Decrease the likelihood of becoming obese or overweight. Replacing high-calorie, high-fat foods with fruits and vegetables can help achieve and maintain a healthy weight. In addition to being relatively low in calories, the significant water and fiber content in fruits and vegetables aids in weight control by helping you feel full, thus reducing your total caloric intake.

Decrease high blood pressure. The potassium and magnesium in fruits and vegetables help to minimize damage to arteries.

Lower the risk of heart disease and stroke. Fruits and vegetables contain potassium and fiber, which decrease hypertension (high blood pressure), a leading cause of heart disease. They also contain vitamin C, which strengthens blood vessels.

Reduce bad cholesterol. The liver produces bile acids out of circulating blood cholesterol. Soluble fiber in fruits and vegetables decreases blood cholesterol by binding with these bile acids and excreting them. The process, in turn, decreases the amount of circulating cholesterol that can lead to atherosclerosis (plaque in the arteries).

Prevent or help control diabetes. The fiber provided in fruits and vegetables helps to control weight and blood sugar levels.

Reduce the risk of cancer. Scientists estimate that 40% to 60% of all cancers are related to what we eat. Antioxidants, which are available in fruits and vegetables, are able to neutralize or minimize the harmful effects of free radicals—products formed when cells use oxygen. Free radicals can damage cells, which can lead to diseases such as cancer.

Promote healthy aging. Fruits and vegetables provide beneficial compounds to keep all of the vital systems in the body working efficiently throughout the years. These compounds may protect against Alzheimer's disease and dementia. They also help to reduce skin wrinkling.

Protect vision. Fruits and vegetables, especially carrots, broccoli, sweet potatoes, squash, red bell peppers, cantaloupe, mango, and dark leafy vegetables, contain beta-carotene, which is specifically associated with delayed development of various forms of cataracts.

Decrease the risk of developing diverticulosis and other gastrointestinal disorders. Many fruits and vegetables provide insoluble fiber that helps maintain normal bowel function, reducing the risk of diverticulosis, and other GI disorders.

Minimize birth defects. Many fruits and vegetables, especially dark green leafy vegetables, citrus fruits, and dried beans, contain folic acid. Folic acid has been shown to decrease the risk of certain types of birth defects.

Source: 2010 Produce for Better Health Foundation.

Summary

To reduce, prevent, or control the chances of getting certain types of cancer, heart disease and/or adult diabetes, and to feel better physically, the consumption of macronutrients for the entire day is represented by the following Nutrition Facts Label.

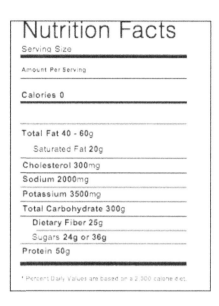

LEVEL 5

Start Early! Age and Caloric Balance

Each individual should maintain the appropriate caloric balance during each stage of life.

* Childhood;
* Adolescence;
* Adulthood;
* Older age.

It is the key to maintaining health and wellness, preventing obesity, and avoiding and/or overcoming chronic diseases. The guidelines that follow give the toolset to adjust macronutrient intake throughout each stage of life.

Source: Dietary Reference Intakes, Nutrition Facts Labels, Institutes of Medicine.

2–3 years: 1,000–1,400 Calorie Intake

Nutrient	Unit of Measure	Daily Totals
Total Fat	grams (g)	30–55
Saturated Fatty Acids	grams (g)	12–16
Cholesterol	milligrams (mg)	< 300
Sodium	milligrams (mg)	1,000–1,500
Potassium	milligrams (mg)	3,500
Total Carbohydrate	grams (g)	110–230
Fiber	grams (g)	14–19
Protein	grams (g)	13

4–8 years: 1,400–1,600 Calorie Intake

Nutrient	Unit of Measure	Daily Totals
Total Fat	grams (g)	39–62
Saturated Fatty Acids	grams (g)	16–18
Cholesterol	milligrams	<300
Sodium	milligrams (mg)	1,200–1,900
Potassium	milligrams (mg)	3,800
Total Carbohydrate	grams (g)	230–260
Fiber	grams (g)	20–25
Protein	grams (g)	20

9–13 years Girls: 1,600–2,000 Calorie Intake

Nutrient	Unit of Measure	Daily Totals
Total Fat	grams (g)	62–85
Saturated Fatty Acids	grams (g)	18–22
Cholesterol	milligrams (mg)	<300
Sodium	milligrams (mg)	1,500–2,200
Potassium	milligrams (mg)	4,500
Total Carbohydrate	grams (g)	180–325
Fiber	grams (g)	23–28
Protein	grams (g)	34

9–13 years Boys: 1,600–2,000 Calorie Intake

Nutrient	Unit of Measure	Daily Totals
Total Fat	grams (g)	62–85
Saturated Fatty Acids	grams (g)	20–25
Cholesterol	milligrams (mg)	<300
Sodium	milligrams (mg)	1,500–2,200
Potassium	milligrams (mg)	4,500
Total Carbohydrate	grams (g)	180–325
Fiber	grams (g)	25–30
Protein	grams (g)	35

14–18 Girls: 2,000 Calorie Intake

Nutrient	Unit of Measure	Daily Totals
Total Fat	grams (g)	55–78
Saturated Fatty Acids	grams (g)	22
Cholesterol	milligrams (mg)	<300
Sodium	milligrams (mg)	1,500–2,300
Potassium	milligrams (mg)	4,500
Total Carbohydrate	grams (g)	225–325
Fiber	grams (g)	23
Protein	grams (g)	46

14–18 Boys: 2,200–2,400 Calorie Intake

Nutrient	Unit of Measure	Daily Totals
Total Fat	grams (g)	61–95
Saturated Fatty Acids	grams (g)	24–27
Cholesterol	milligrams (mg)	<300
Sodium	milligrams (mg)	1,500–2,300
Potassium	milligrams (mg)	4,500
Total Carbohydrate	grams (g)	250–390
Fiber	grams (g)	31–34
Protein	grams (g)	52

Adults: 2,000 Calorie Intake

Nutrient	Unit of Measure	Daily Totals
Total Fat	grams (g)	65
Saturated Fatty Acids	grams (g)	20
Cholesterol	milligrams (mg)	300
Sodium	milligrams (mg)	2,400
Potassium	milligrams (mg)	3,500
Total Carbohydrate	grams (g)	300
Fiber	grams (g)	25
Protein	grams (g)	50

Summary

For your convenience, **Level 5** provides the daily recommended intake of macronutrients by age and gender to readily adapt to each member of the family.

LEVEL 6

The Complete Nutrition Facts Label

Level 2 Explains the <u>macronutrient</u> information on the Nutrition Facts Label. But Nutrition Facts Labels also have standards for <u>micronutrients</u> or <u>vitamins and minerals</u>. These food components have specific functions in the body and all of them together are required for overall health. The complete listing follows and is based on a 2000-calorie daily intake.

1. <u>Macro</u>nutrients & <u>Micro</u>nutrients (Vitamins and Minerals)

Macronutrient	**Unit of Measure**	**Daily Values**
Total Fat	grams (g)	65
Saturated Fatty Acids	grams (g)	20
Cholesterol	milligrams (mg)	300
Sodium	milligrams (mg)	2,400
Potassium	milligrams (mg)	3,500
Total Carbohydrate	grams (g)	300
Fiber	grams (g)	25
Protein	grams (g)	50
Micronutrient	**Unit of Measure**	**Daily Values**
Vitamin A	International Unit (IU)	5,000
Vitamin C	milligrams (mg)	60
Calcium	milligrams (mg)	1,000
Iron	milligrams (mg)	18
Vitamin D	International Unit (IU)	400
Vitamin E	International Unit (IU)	30
Vitamin K	micrograms (μg)	80.0

Micronutrient	Unit of Measure	Daily Values
Thiamin	milligrams (mg)	1.5
Riboflavin	milligrams (mg)	1.7
Niacin	milligrams (mg)	20.0
Vitamin B_6	milligrams (mg)	2.0
Folate	micrograms (µg)	400.0
Vitamin B_{12}	micrograms (µg)	6.0
Biotin	micrograms (µg)	300.0
Pantothenic Acid	milligrams (mg)	10.0
Phosphorus	milligrams (mg)	1,000.0
Iodine	micrograms (µg)	150.0
Magnesium	milligrams (mg)	400.0
Zinc	milligrams (mg)	15.0
Selenium	micrograms (µg)	70.0
Copper	milligrams (mg)	2.0
Manganese	milligrams (mg)	2.0
Chromium	micrograms (µg)	120.0
Molybdenum	micrograms (µg)	75.0
Chloride	milligrams (mg)	3,400.0

2. Combining the Label Information: Calculating the Amount(s) of Vitamins and Minerals Per Serving

Nutrition Facts

Serving Size: About (20g)
Servings Per Container: 16

	Amount Per Serving	% Daily Value*
Total Calories	60	
Calories From Fat	15	
Total Fat	2 g	3%
Saturated Fat	1 g	4%
Trans Fat	0 g	
Cholesterol	0 mg	0%
Sodium	45 mg	2%
Total Carbohydrates	15 g	5%
Dietary Fiber	4 g	17%
Sugars	4 g	
Sugar Alcohols (Polyols)	3 g	
Protein	2 g	
Vitamin A		0%
Vitamin C		0%
Calcium		2%
Iron		2%

*Percent Daily Values are based on a 2,000 calorie diet.

Ingredients: Wheat flour, unsweetened chocolate, erythritol, inulin, oat flour, cocoa powder, evaporated cane juice, whey protein concentrate, corn starch (low glycemic), natural flavors, salt, baking soda, wheat gluten, guar gum

Calculation 1: The amount of Iron in a serving of the product is 2% of what is desired for total daily consumption. The Complete Nutrition Facts Label gives the amount of Iron for total daily consumption as 18mg (see page 81). When combining the label information (18mg × 2%), the amount of Iron in a serving is 0.36 mg.

Calculation 2: The amount of Calcium in a serving of the product is 2% of what is desired for total daily consumption. The Complete Nutrition Facts Label gives the amount of Calcium for total daily consumption as 1,000mg (see page 81). When combining the label information (1,000mg × 2%), the amount of Calcium in a serving is 20 mg.

3. Examining the Ingredients Listed at the Bottom of the Label for:

Nutrition Facts

Serving Size: About (20g)
Servings Per Container: 16

	Amount Per Serving	% Daily Value*
Total Calories	60	
Calories From Fat	15	
Total Fat	2 g	3%
Saturated Fat	1 g	4%
Trans Fat	0 g	
Cholesterol	0 mg	0%
Sodium	45 mg	2%
Total Carbohydrates	15 g	5%
Dietary Fiber	4 g	17%
Sugars	4 g	
Sugar Alcohols (Polyols)	3 g	
Protein	2 g	
Vitamin A		0%
Vitamin C		0%
Calcium		2%
Iron		2%

*Percent Daily Values are based on a 2,000 calorie diet.

Ingredients: Wheat flour, unsweetened chocolate, erythritol, inulin, oat flour, cocoa powder, evaporated cane juice, whey protein concentrate, corn starch (low glycemic), natural flavors, salt, baking soda, wheat gluten, guar gum

* Food allergies, i.e. gluten
* Added sugars: See **Level 1 Rule 5** on page 13–15.
* Ingredients to avoid

Most nutritionists and medical professionals believe that products with long or chemical-sounding words among the ingredients should be avoided. Examples include:

Artificial colors and flavorings - azo dyes and FD&C US certified food colorings—including Yellow 5, Yellow 6, Red 3, Red 40, Blue 1, Blue 2, Green 3, and Orange B

Monosodium glutamate (MSG), also known as hydrolyzed vegetable protein, hydrolyzed protein, hydrolyzed plant/vegetable protein (HVP), hydrolyzed milk protein; modified food starch, plant protein extract, sodium caseinate, calcium caseinate, autolyzed yeast extract, textured protein, hydrolyzed oat flour, etc., partially hydrogenated oils—trans fat

Chemical preservatives including benzoic acid; BHA (butylated hydroxy-anisole), BHT (butylated hydroxy-toluene), calcium disodium EDTA, disodium phosphate, disodium guanylate, disodium inosinate, EDTA, potassium bromate, bisulfate, dihydrogen citrate, propyl gallate, sodium benzoate, sodium bisulfate, sodium caseinate,

sodium hydroxide, sodium nitrate, sodium nitrite, sulfur dioxide, TBHQ (tertiary butylhydroquinone)

Highly-processed refined sugars including corn sweeteners, corn syrups, corn syrupsolids, high fructose corn syrup

Artificial sweeteners including acesulfame potassium, acesulfame-K, aspartame (NutraSweet or Equal), cyclamate, neotame, saccharin (Sweet'n Low), sucralose (Splenda)

Refined grains including brominated flour, bleached flour, enriched flour, white flour

Diglycerides, monoglycerides, and phosphoric acids

Products "enriched" with vitamins or minerals, which indicates that they are more processed.

Summary

This completes **Level 6** of nutrition as a basic skill. These are the final "how-to's" of interpreting food labels.

LEVEL 7

Reality Checks!

Step 1: Know Your Healthy Weight

Achieving and/or maintaining a healthy body weight is a crucial destination for good health! Find your ideal weight and make it one of your goals to achieve health and wellness.

Weight Chart for Men

Height	Small Frame	Medium Frame	Large Frame
5'2"	128–134	131–141	138–150
5'3"	130–136	133–143	140–153
5'4"	132–138	135–145	142–156
5'5"	134–140	137–148	144–160
5'6"	136–142	139–151	146–164
5'7"	138–145	142–154	149–168
5'8"	140–148	145–157	152–172
5'9"	142–151	148–160	155–176
5'10"	144–154	151–163	158–180
5'11"	146–157	154–166	161–184
6'0"	149–160	157–170	164–188
6'1"	152–164	160–174	168–192
6'2"	155–168	164–178	172–197
6'3"	158–172	167–182	176–202
6'4"	162–176	171–187	181–207

Achieving and/or maintaining a healthy body weight is a crucial destination for good health! Find your ideal weight and make it one of your goals to achieve health and wellness.

Weight Chart for Women

Height	Small Frame	Medium Frame	Large Frame
4'10"	102–111	109–121	118–131
4'11"	103–113	111–123	120–134
5'0"	104–115	113–126	122–137
5'1"	106–118	115–129	125–140
5'2"	108–121	118–132	128–143
5'3"	111–124	121–135	131–147
5'4"	114–127	124–138	134–151
5'5"	117–130	127–141	137–155
5'6"	120–133	130–144	140–159
5'7"	123–136	133–147	143–163
5'8"	126–139	136–150	146–167
5'9"	129–142	139–153	149–170
5'10"	132–145	142–156	152–173
5'11"	135–148	145–159	155–176
6' 0"	138–151	148–162	158–179

Step 2: Know the Waist-Height Relationship

The waist to height ratio. Waistlines should be no more than half of an individual's height. Keeping your waist circumference to less than half of your height can help prevent the onset of conditions like stroke, heart disease and diabetes. It can also add years to your life.

Step 3: Know Your Body Mass Index (BMI) and What It Means

Body Mass Index (BMI) is another crucial destination for good health!

Height	Minimal Risk (BMI Under 25)	Overweight (BMI 25.0–29.9)	Obese (BMI 30.0 and Above)
4′10″	118 lb or less	119–142 lb	143 lb or more
4′11″	123	124–147	148
5′0″	127	128–152	153
5′1″	131	132–157	158
5′2″	135	136–163	164
5′3″	140	141–168	169
5′4″	144	145–173	174
5′5″	149	150–179	180
5′6″	154	155–185	186
5′7″	158	159–190	191
5′8″	163	164–196	197
5′9″	168	169–202	203
5′10″	173	174–208	209
5′11″	178	179–214	215
6′0″	183	184–220	221
6′1″	188	189–226	227
6′2″	193	194–232	233
6′3″	199	200–239	240
6′4″	204	205–245	246

Source: The American Heart Association.

What Does BMI Mean?

Normal weight: BMI = 18.5–24.9
Overweight: BMI = 25–29.9
Obese: BMI = 30 or greater

Step 4: Become Familiar with Individual Caloric Needs Based on Age, Gender and Physical Activity Level

Gender/ Activity level[b]	Male/ Sedentary	Male/ Moderately Active	Male/ Active	Female[c]/ Sedentary	Female[c]/ Moderately Active	Female[c]/ Active
Age (years)						
2	1,000	1,000	1,000	1,000	1,000	1,000
3	1,200	1,400	1,400	1,000	1,200	1,400
4	1,200	1,400	1,600	1,200	1,400	1,400
5	1,200	1,400	1,600	1,200	1,400	1,600
6	1,400	1,600	1,800	1,200	1,400	1,600
7	1,400	1,600	1,800	1,200	1,600	1,800
8	1,400	1,600	2,000	1,400	1,600	1,800
9	1,600	1,800	2,000	1,400	1,600	1,800
10	1,600	1,800	2,200	1,400	1,800	2,000
11	1,800	2,000	2,200	1,600	1,800	2,000
12	1,800	2,200	2,400	1,600	2,000	2,200
13	2,000	2,200	2,600	1,600	2,000	2,200
14	2,000	2,400	2,800	1,800	2,000	2,400
15	2,200	2,600	3,000	1,800	2,000	2,400
16	2,400	2,800	3,200	1,800	2,000	2,400
17	2,400	2,800	3,200	1,800	2,000	2,400
18	2,400	2,800	3,200	1,800	2,000	2,400
19-20	2,600	2,800	3,000	2,000	2,200	2,400
21-25	2,400	2,800	3,000	2,000	2,200	2,400
26-30	2,400	2,600	3,000	1,800	2,000	2,400
31-35	2,400	2,600	3,000	1,800	2,000	2,200
36-40	2,400	2,600	2,800	1,800	2,000	2,200
41-45	2,200	2,600	2,800	1,800	2,000	2,200
46-50	2,200	2,400	2,800	1,800	2,000	2,200
51-55	2,200	2,400	2,800	1,600	1,800	2,200
56-60	2,200	2,400	2,600	1,600	1,800	2,200
61-65	2,000	2,400	2,600	1,600	1,800	2,000
66-70	2,000	2,200	2,600	1,600	1,800	2,000
71-75	2,000	2,200	2,600	1,600	1,800	2,000
76+	2,000	2,200	2,400	1,600	1,800	2,000

Sedentary means a lifestyle that includes only light physical activity that is associated with typical day-to-day life.

Moderately active means a lifestyle that includes physical activity that is equivalent to walking about 1.5 to 3 miles per day at 3 to 4 miles per hour, in addition to light physical activity that is associated with typical day-to-day life.

Active means a lifestyle that includes physical activity that is equivalent to walking more than 3 miles per day at 3 to 4 miles per hour, in addition to the light physical activity that is associated with typical day-to-day life.

Source: Britten/Marcoe/Yamini/Development of Food Intake Patterns for the MyPyramid Food Guidance System.

Step 5: Become Physically Active—Physical Activity Guidelines

6 to 17 years..................Children and adolescents should do 60 minutes (1 hour) or more of physical activity daily.

* Aerobic: Most of the 60 or more minutes for each day should be spent engaging in either moderate- or vigorous-intensity aerobic physical activity and should include vigorous-intensity physical activity at least 3 days a week.

* Muscle-strengthening: As part of their 60 or more minutes of daily physical activity, children and adolescents should include muscle-strengthening physical activity at least 3 days a week.

* Bone-strengthening: As part of their 60 or more minutes of daily physical activity, children and adolescents should include bone-strengthening physical activity at least 3 days a week.

18 to 64 years................All adults should avoid inactivity! Some physical activity is better than none, and adults who participate in any amount of physical activity gain some health benefits.

* For substantial health benefits, adults should do at least 150 minutes (2 hours and 30 minutes) a week of moderate-intensity physical activity, or 75 minutes (1 hour and 15 minutes) a week of vigorous-intensity aerobic physical activity or an equivalent combination of the two. Aerobic activity should be performed in episodes of at least 10 minutes, and preferably, it should be spread throughout the week.

* For additional and more extensive health benefits, adults should increase their aerobic physical activity to 300 minutes (5 hours) a week of moderate-intensity aerobic physical activity, or 150 minutes a week of vigorous-intensity aerobic physical activity, or an equivalent combination of the two. Additional health benefits are gained by engaging in physical activity beyond this amount.

* Adults should also include muscle-strengthening activities that involve all major muscle groups on 2 or more days a week.

65 years and older ....Older adults should follow the adult guidelines. When older adults cannot meet the adult guidelines, they should be as physically active as their abilities and conditions will allow.

   * Older adults should do exercises that maintain or improve balance if they are at risk of falling.

   * Older adults should determine their level of effort for physical activity relative to their level of fitness.

   * Older adults with chronic conditions should understand whether and how their conditions affect their ability to do regular physical activity safely.

a) *Moderate-intensity physical activity*: Aerobic activity that increases a person's heart rate and breathing to some extent. On a scale relative to a person's capacity, moderate-intensity activity is usually a 5 or 6 on a 0 to 10 scale. Brisk walking, dancing, swimming, and bicycling on a level terrain are examples.

b) *Vigorous-intensity physical activity*: Aerobic activity that greatly increases a person's heart rate and breathing. On a scale relative to a person's capacity, vigorous-intensity activity is usually a 7 or 8 on a 0 to 10 scale. Jogging, singles tennis, swimming continuous laps, and bicycling uphill are examples.

c) *Muscle-strengthening activity*: Physical activity including exercises that increase skeletal muscle strength, power, endurance, and mass. It includes strength training, resistance training, muscular strength, and endurance exercises.

d) *Bone-strengthening activity*: Physical activity that produces an impact or tension force on bones, which promotes bone growth and strength. Running, jumping rope, and lifting weights are examples.

Source: U.S. Department of Health and Human Services.

Step 6: Understand the Results of Medical Tests

Blood Pressure

Normal:	Less than 120/80 mmHg
Prehypertension:	120/80 to 139/89 mmHg
Hypertension:	140/90 or higher mmHg

Cholesterol

Total Cholesterol

Desirable:	Less than 200 mg/dl
Borderline high:	200–239 mg/dl
High:	240 mg/dl and above

LDL Cholesterol

Optimal:	Less than 100 mg/dl
Near optimal:	100–129 mg/dl
Borderline high:	130–159 mg/dl
High:	160–189 mg/dl
Very high:	190 mg/dl and above

HDL Cholesterol

An HDL of less than 40 mg/dl is a major risk factor for heart disease.

Blood Glucose

Normal:	Under 99 mg/dl
Prediabetes:	100–125 mg/dl
Diabetes:	126 mg/dl and above

Source: U.S. Department of Health and Human Services.

Conclusion

Utilize these tools to take the first steps in assessing your health and wellness. If need be, begin setting goals and preparing for new behaviors as you consult with medical professionals.

LEVEL 8

The 95% of Claims That "You Don't Need To Know"

Food labels use lots of terms and jargon including "fortified", "refined", "lower in sodium", "lower in saturated fat", "no fat", "low calorie", "low-fat", "zero cholesterol", "lite" and more! But who knows or can keep track of what these ambiguous terms mean? More so, who wants to remember the definitions of all of the terms? You'd continuously need a guide on hand to find out what each claim really means! But "you don't need to know" or worry about all the claims because most of them are based on the same ten numbers that you have memorized from **LEVEL 2**!

The goal of this level is simply to bring clarity and "reinforce" the process by which this manual makes navigating the guidelines of nutrition easier for anyone and everyone. This process forms the premise of "you don't need to know!"

Reinforcement 1

If You Know . . .
    Total fat = 65g daily,

Then You <u>Don't</u> Need To Know . . .
    Fat free..............Less than 0.5g of fat per serving
    Low fat..............3g of fat or less
    Reduced fat........At least 25 percent less fat per serving than the regular version
    Lean..................Less than 10g of fat, 4.5g of saturated fat, and 95mg of cholesterol
    Extra lean..........Less than 5g of fat, 2g of saturated fat, and 95mg of cholesterol
    Light or lite ....At least 1/3 fewer calories or no more than half the fat of the regular
                        product, or no more than half the sodium of the regular product.

Reinforcement 2

If You Know . . .
    Saturated fat = 20g daily,

Then You <u>Don't</u> Need To Know . . .
    Zero trans fat ....Less than 0.5g per serving
    Low in saturated fat........1g or less of saturated fat per serving.

Reinforcement 3

If You Know . . .
    Cholesterol = 300mg daily,

Then You <u>Don't</u> Need To Know . . .
    Cholesterol-free .... Less than 2mg of cholesterol and no more than 2g of saturated fat per serving
    Zero cholesterol .... Less than 2mg of cholesterol and no more than 2g of saturated fat per serving
    Low cholesterol .... 20 or fewer mg of cholesterol and 2g or less of saturated fat
    Reduced cholesterol ...... At least 25 percent less cholesterol than the regular product and 2g or less of saturated fat.

Reinforcement 4

If You Know . . .
    Sodium = 2,400mg (one teaspoon) daily,

Then You <u>Don't</u> Need To Know . . .
    Sodium free or salt free .... Less than 5mg of sodium per serving
    Very low sodium .... 35mg or less per serving
    Low sodium .... 140mg or less per serving
    Low sodium meal .... 140mg or less per 3½ ounces
    Reduced or less sodium .... At least 25 percent less per serving than the regular version
    Unsalted or no salt added .... No salt added during processing.

Reinforcement 5

If You Know . . .
    Potassium = 3,500mg daily,

Then You <u>Don't</u> Need To Know . . .
    . . . any other claims. Just ensure that for a 2,000-calorie daily diet, you consume approximately 3,500mg of potassium per day.

Reinforcement 6

If You Know . . .
    Total carbohydrates = 300g daily

Then You <u>Don't</u> Need To Know . . .
    . . . any other claims. Just ensure that for a 2,000-calorie daily diet, you consume approximately 300g of carbohydrates per day.

Reinforcement 7

If You Know . . .
> Dietary fiber = 25g daily,

Then You <u>Don't</u> Need To Know . . .
> . . . any other claims. Just ensure that for a 2,000-calorie daily diet, you consume at least 25g of fiber per day.

Reinforcement 8

If You Know . . .
> Protein = 50g daily,

Then You <u>Don't</u> Need To Know . . .
> . . . any other claims. Just ensure that for a 2,000-calorie daily diet, you consume at least 50g of protein per day.

Reinforcement 9

If You Know . . .
> The amount of each macronutrient to be consumed daily,

Then You <u>Don't</u> Need To Know . . .

Calorie-free	Less than 5 calories per serving
Low calorie	40 calories or less per serving
Reduced or less calories	At least 25 percent fewer calories per serving than the regular version
Light or "lite"	1/3 of the calories per serving than the regular version
Light	A nutritionally altered product contains 1/3 fewer calories or half the fat of the reference food
Light	Sodium content of a low-calorie, low-fat food has been reduced by 50 percent
Light	Can be used to describe texture and color, as long as the label explains the intent for using the term
Reduced	A nutritionally altered product contains at least 25 percent less of a nutrient or of calories than the regular or reference product
Less/fewer	A food, whether altered or not, contains 25 percent less of a nutrient or of calories than the reference food
More	A serving of food, whether altered or not, contains a nutrient that is at least 10 percent more of the daily value than the reference food. The 10 percent of daily value also applies to "fortified", "enriched", "added", "extra" and "plus" claims, but the food must be altered.

Reinforcement 10

If You Know . . .

The sugar standards:

Women should consume no more than 6 teaspoons (24g) of added sugar daily

Men should consume no more than 9 teaspoons (36g) of added sugar daily

Children under 12 should consume no more than 3 teaspoons (12g) of added sugar per day

Then You <u>Don't</u> Need To Know . . .

Sugar-free...................................Less than 0.5g of sugar per serving or calories per serving

Reduced sugar or less sugar ....At least 25 percent less sugar per serving compared to an appropriate reference food

Sugar-free...................................Less than 0.5g of sugar per serving

No added sugars........................No sugar or sugar-containing ingredient such as juice or dry fruit is added during processing

Low sugar ....Not defined as a claim on food labels.

Summary

This level demonstrates the scope and depth of what makes nutrition complicated. We hope you realize that now that you have learned the ten recommended daily amounts for the macronutrients from **Level 2**, you have eliminated the need to focus on more than 95% of nutritional labeling!

REINFORCEMENT

The Complete Guide to Developing Nutrition Skills is intended to be an eye-opener of nutritional information that aids in leading healthy lives, addressing gaps in nutritional knowledge, and executing smarter solutions to health challenges.

We believe that the current diet should be the starting point for the analysis of food intake. It provides a familiar foundation to build upon and is the most logical method to gain the skills needed to achieve nutritional adequacy. On day one, we suggest that you begin examining your food intake (the macronutrients) and, if need be, begin maneuvering and making adjustments from that point. Too many times, we approach nutrition and dieting by "scrapping" most, if not all, foods in our current diets. But we must begin the journey from the point of familiarity. Simply put, it's about bridge crossing, traveling from where we are to where we need to be.

In this one document, we have provided the route to travel, for we all must be proactive and seek nutritional excellence!

CPSIA information can be obtained at www.ICGtesting.com
Printed in the USA
BVOW11s1111260415

397734BV00004B/6/P